Surviving Life After a Heart Attack

Advice from a Fellow Patient

By Richard Snider

Dedication

To Dr. Anne Safko
– thank you.

Prologue

OK, you've survived. Now what?

I'm not a doctor so there's no medical advice. I'm not a nutritionist so there's no dietary advice – except stop eating triple cheeseburgers. And I'm not a cleric, so I'm not talking about which church to visit.

Trust me, there are plenty of people who will offer all this advice and more whether you want it or not.

This is a story of someone just like you. I went through a major heart attack on Sept. 4, 2002. The kind that kills 19 of every 20 men, my doc says. I'm the one who survived. Yeah, think about that for a moment. Heavy.

This book is merely advice from someone who has walked your path for the last 12 years. All your family and friends are well meaning, but unless they've been through it they can't understand. It's the same with everything: losing your job, becoming an empty nester or enduring a health crisis – unless you've been there, the words lack strength.

This is my story. This is my advice and I hope it saves you a few steps in the journey to recovery. It's a short story because you're probably not up for a long sermon; just some friendly advice.

So before we begin, let me say this:

One day, you're going to be all right. You'll be playing with your grandkids, throwing the ball to the dog, fishing, going to the ballgames.

It's a journey that doesn't happen overnight. But, today is a step towards that day when life is good once more. Just keep heading towards it. Don't give up. Don't despair. Stay positive. Be strong.

Because you can do it.

Table of Contents

1

The first days

If you're reading this, you're probably out of the hospital and sitting on your couch.

Please get up.

I know you're scared and you have a right to be scared. You just survived a heart attack.

You just want to be left alone. No doctors poking you. No visitors looking scared. No wondering if you're going to die. You just want to sit in your favorite chair and watch TV in peace. Let the talk of a strict diet and exercise and lifestyle changes stay away for awhile.

I'm with you there. But as long as doctors approve, you need to walk around some. Clear your head. Enjoy being alive.

Just breathe.

You don't need to make a thousand changes at once or a thousand decisions right now. You need to just breathe. Let your mind and body rest. But, do get off the couch. Sound contradictory? Get used to that.

2

Dealing with well wishers

In the first few days after returning home, I received calls, emails and cards from 125 people. It was overwhelming. And, I stupidly tried to respond.

When I needed open heart surgery 17 months later to finally correct that troublesome artery, I told everyone not to call or email me. I would have my daughters send out daily mass emails on my progress and get back to people when I could.

It made all the difference. You really need peace and quiet. The phone bothered me because I knew it was someone wanting to talk to me and I just didn't feel up to it for awhile.

I always wrestled with this thought: thank you for caring about me. It means a lot. But, please understand it upsets me that I can't respond right now – so let me reach out when I'm ready.

It's OK to be selfish right now. People will understand and wait for word. Having someone send out chain emails will suffice for now.

One day, when you feel like a quick conversation, pick up the phone and call someone. The next day, call someone else. Ask them to send emails to everyone on what you discussed.

In a week or two, have a friend or two come by for lunch. You may feel up to going out for an hour, so it works for both sides. They'll even pick up the tab.

You're looking for that normalcy in your life once more and that's a good sign. Two weeks after open heart surgery, I just sat in my car. I wasn't allowed to drive, but just sitting in the driver's seat with the window rolled down and the radio on felt so good.

You need someone in your life to act as a gatekeeper. Otherwise, you'll wear yourself out. Take small steps every day to resuming your life, but don't be in too big of a rush to return to the grind. Once you show up at work, everyone will say take it easy — but expect you to be 100 percent again. Like I said, there are lots of mixed signals in recovery.

People often gave me books and videos, saying they wish they had a few weeks off. Now I could enjoy reading and movies. What they don't understand is you're mentally fried. That pile of books only serves as a reminder of what you can't do right now and will further frustrate you. I don't think I ever watched those movies or read those books.

I eventually gave them all away. It's OK to ignore them.

I enjoyed the fruit baskets, though. I still have one basket for my medications. Just don't expect any baskets of sausage and cheese.

3

Make no rash decisions

Are you going to retire, people asked. I was 42 years old working 80-hour weeks as a sports writer for a Washington, D.C. daily newspaper. I was certainly too young to retire (and too poor) and was shocked people asked me that.

So what was I going to do now? Actually, it's OK to do nothing right now.

Maybe a heart attack is a time to reflect on your life. Perhaps it's time to do whatever you've been waiting to do. A new job. A new love. A new passion.

Or maybe it's just a pause button and you go back to what you were doing – minus unhealthy habits like smoking, drugs, excessive alcohol use and eating spam out of cans.

It's OK to do nothing. It doesn't mean midlife crisis time. If you're happy with your life, keep going. Don't feel guilty for doing so. Not everybody becomes a different person.

So don't make any rash decisions, please. Give yourself time to heal mentally and physically. Three months for some, six months for others, maybe a year for you.

It's OK, there's no clock on making decisions.

But, don't decide you have to make a life change because of the heart attack. In time if you want to change things, then go ahead. Just remember, there's nobody saying you need to but yourself.

4

God, where are you?

In the past 12 years, I have grown from someone who believed in God to someone who realizes God loves me, too.

I'm not in the front row of church every Sunday, but God is in my thoughts and hopefully deeds every day. I know God has carried me through some tough times.

Perhaps the most clear moment of it all came shortly before I was wheeled into open-heart surgery. I had been through

17 months of hell and knew this was the key moment.

I told my wife not to worry.

"Either I'm going to wake up to see you and everything will be all right," I said, "or I will wake up to see God and everything will be all right. But either way, this ends now and only better times lie ahead."

Funny what morphine does to you.

But seriously, I knew things would be OK. That I knew God would see me through.

So you're wondering why God has somehow abandoned you? You're a good person. You don't hurt other people. You've tried to live a good life. So why is this happening to you? Why isn't God protecting you?

I can't answer that.

Well, actually, I think my answer would be God hasn't abandoned you. Maybe it's the other way. Maybe you haven't given yourself over to God?

Now, I'm not saying God is punishing you. Nor am I saying repent and become a monk. God has all the monks he wants. He needs you to be you.

So take a deep breath and realize we're human beings. Our bodies break down and nobody truly gets out alive. We all want more time and pray for a healthy life.

I'm not a cleric, but my advice is to think more about God in your life because God is thinking about you.

Postscript: This story is true and too funny to pass up telling. After I came out of surgery, I saw my wife and smiled. The surgeon came over and I said, "Doc . . ."

I couldn't utter much, given the meds and all. I was the second of eight open heart operations he was performing that day so he only had a moment.

"OK, no golf for three months," he said.

What?

"I'm not kidding, no golf for three months."

Wait — how am I? Was the surgery a success? I'm trying to escape the fog to simply ask if I'm all right?

"OK, if you want to putt after a month, go ahead."

Who are you, the PGA Tour doctor? Repeat after me, Doc: "You're OK."

He laughed and said I was fine. What I didn't realize was in his mind I was already headed for recovery. But seriously, Doc: start off with that sentence.

Maybe his clientele was old guys on golf courses. I tried to learn the game after my heart attack. Everybody said I needed a hobby. I found golf boring. But, I did go to the golf range three months later and the doc was right — swinging that club is hell on your chest.

5

Go for a walk

When your doctor says it's OK to exercise, don't buy a gym membership right away. You'll go for a few weeks and probably quit.

Instead, just go for a walk. Take someone with you at first if you feel unsteady. Have your cell phone just in case.

But the road back to good health begins with the first step. Walk whatever pace you like. It's not a race or even timed overall. You're just getting some fresh air, a little exercise and clearing your mind.

Listen to the birds. I did that so often as a kid and got away from it. Now I try to slow down when I'm out in the yard and the birds are chirping, trying to tell me to live in the moment.

Maybe you make it down to the corner on the first day. A week later, another corner. Then a mile. Maybe once a day, maybe twice. Eventually, take the dog with you if it's not too straining.

I walked on neighborhood recycling days. You'd be amazed how many cans you'll pick up and throw in the next bin you see.

But, I also learned when local school bus pickups were because I was tired of parents looking hard at some stranger walking by their kids. I totally understand. I'd be the same way if I were them. So, I just wait until the buses are gone and avoid the dirty looks.

Just walk. Do something you like. It's important to get off the couch.

6

Rehab is worth it

Your doctor may ask if you'd like to go to rehabilitation classes three months after your heart attack.

Absolutely.

Think of it as a gym with nurses and a heart monitor. It's just treadmills, exercise bikes and such. You pedal and walk around at your pace for one hour, then listen to someone talk for a few minutes after improving your health.

The real benefit is meeting others going through the same thing as you. Nobody understands better than those enduring the same problems, fears, concerns and limits.

You'll feel better talking about it. You'll learn from others. Think of it as AA for heart patients.

"Hello, I'm Rick and I'm a heart attack survivor. It has been X days since my heart attack."

Yeah, sounds weird, but it will help. Like I said earlier, nobody understands better what you're going through than fellow heart attack survivors. Maybe you'll help others, too.

7

Find your passion

What do you really care about most?

It's not a simple answer. But once you get past the classic line of *family*, ask yourself once more.

What do really care about the most?

And then the silence is deafening. We're so used to the everyday rut of life that we don't often have a moment to think about our greatest passion — much less do it.

But the heart attack gives you time to pause and hit a reset button. I said earlier not to make any rash decisions. This is a long-term thought on how to regroup. Depending on your age and whether you're working or retired will impact the answer, of course.

But what do you really care about the most? The answer won't come in a flash. It may not come soon, but keep thinking about it because one day you'll have an answer.

It took me a few years before deciding my greatest interest is traveling. I've been to 14 countries on three continents and just enjoy seeing different places. I've learned that in the end people are all pretty much the same, but the beauty of their lives and their surroundings can be so emotionally fulfilling.

Maybe you've worked in an office all your life and now just want to be outside. There are a lot of jobs, part-time and voluntary, that can release you. Don't worry about how much it pays, but how rewarding it is.

Same with helping others. Volunteering is so rewarding. Maybe you're raising money for a cause, helping local food drives, tutoring students, mentoring kids, working at a library, saving animals in a rescue shelter or serving as an usher in church. There are many ways to enjoy your time.

8

The rest of the story

I have come to learn one very true thing since the heart attack: It may not be where I want to go, but God takes me where I need to be.

What does that mean? I've spent many an hour reflecting upon it. And one day sitting in a Chicago hotel room waiting to cover a ballgame, I felt God speak to me.

"Be happy wherever you are," He said.

Now I know you're thinking I'm nuts. That I crossed a line. God spoke to me?

Well, I really don't care if you believe it or not. I believe it and why not? I'm a son of God. I'm worthy of his love.

And so are you.

My life has changed so much since the heart attack. First, I haven't had a bad day since open heart. Not one day in a hospital. I feel pretty blessed on that point.

In 2005, I moved from reporter to columnist at another newspaper. I needed the change. Reporting is 24/7, especially now with the Internet. Column writing is more analytical and reflective, much like my life is now.

I also became a tour guide in 2010, which came in handy when my newspaper laid off 100 of us in 2013. Nobody wants a 50-plus writer on their payroll that only wants to work 50 hours weekly and wouldn't mind weekends and holidays off. So, I combine writing part-time, tour guiding and other pursuits.

I find myself not really caring about what other people think anymore. That probably comes more from age, but really 99 percent of what we worry about doesn't matter and the other 1 percent will happen anyway.

Forgiving people brings freedom from negative emotions. Understanding few things are really a big deal is freeing. Accepting others are different means everything is fine.

I prayed for God to let me see my children graduate high school, then college and last year to walk each down the aisle for their weddings. Now, every day is a gift. That's why they call it the present.

So after reading this short book, I hope you realize the following: You're free to live your life. Things will be OK.

Now go enjoy life however you'd like.

About the Author

Richard Snider is a journalist and tour guide in Washington, D.C. who survived a heart attack in 2002. His blog MonumentalThoughts.com discusses Washington's history and future. He's also on Twitter: @Snide_Remarks.

www.ingramcontent.com/pod-product-compliance
Lightning Source LLC
Chambersburg PA
CBHW070241290526
45789CB00004B/1719